5:2 FAST DIET
BEGINNERS

25 BEGINNERS LOW CARB RECIPES FOR EASY WEIGHT LOSS WITH THE 5:2 DIET AND PALEO STYLE

J.S. WEST

[FREE eBook LIMITED offer]

As a "Thank You" note to your interest in my recipe books, I'd like to offer my latest eBook for free up to 1000 amazon kindle downloads.
There aren't many left so grab your free copy now!

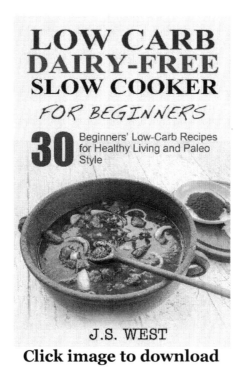

Click image to download

[JOIN FOR FREE]

TABLE OF CONTENTS

Introduction

Chapter 1 - What Is The 5:2 Diet?

Chapter 2 - 5:2 and the Paleo Diet

Chapter 3 - Fast Day Breakfasts

  Soft Boiled Egg

  Scrambled Eggs with Mushrooms

  Spinach Omelette

  Porridge

  Ham Omelette

Chapter 4 - Fast Day Lunches

  Chicken Pita Pockets

  Spring Soup

  Potatoes and Shoots

  Bean Salad

  Tarka Dhal

  Steak Salad

  Artichoke Tortilla

  Miso Soup with Chicken

  Shrimp Salad

Chapter 5 - Fast Day Dinners

  Tomato Shrimp

  Eggplant

  Chow Mein

Squash Tortilla

Ratatouille

Spiced Squash

Fish Burger

Balti

Mediterranean Chili

Thai Chicken

Moroccan Tomatoes

Chapter 6 - One Month of Fasting Day Suggestions

Conclusion

Other Books from J.S. West

I want to thank you and congratulate you for downloading the book, *"5:2 PALEO DIETING FOR BEGINNERS: 25 BEGINNERS LOW CARB RECIPES FOR EASY WEIGHT LOSS WITH THE 5:2 DIET AND PALEO STYLE"*.

This book contains proven steps and strategies on how to lose weight quickly and easily by following the 5:2 diet and paleo style diet in combination with each other.

You will lose at least a pound a week by following the diet plan outlined in this book. After reading this book, you will be armed with the information you need to adopt a combination of 5:2 dieting and paleo dieting in your day to day life. This book also provides you with plenty of delicious and simple recipes to help you make the transition without ever realizing you are even on a diet!

Thanks again for downloading this book, I hope you enjoy it!

Chapter 1 - What Is The 5:2 Diet?

The 5:2 diet is slowly gaining more and more popularity as people come to realize that there is something useful to it. Unfortunately, many people still do not realize just how useful this diet can be. It is also referred to as the Fasting Diet, which is a term that puts many people off from the beginning, before they even have any information about this style of dieting. However, there is no need to fear! You will still be able to eat, and eat well, while following a 5:2 diet.

Simply put, the 5:2 diet works on the principal that you should eat for five days and fast for two. On the five days when you eat, you are able to eat nearly anything you want. You can feel free to load up on calories without worrying too much about how many you are consuming. On the two fasting days, however, women should only eat 500 calories, and men should only eat 600 calories. This is enough caloric intake to keep your body functioning normally and healthily, but it is not going to bloat you or keep your digestive system too backed up.

It can be difficult to mentally handle the concept of fasting for two days, especially when you are first starting out on the 5:2 diet. It sounds much worse than it really is! You are able to choose the two days each week when you fast, and you can change the days depending on your schedule and needs, as long as you have at least two fasting days in a given week. This mean that you are never more than 24 hours away from being able to eat something delicious again. Since your non-fasting days allow basically any kind of food, it is much easier to convince yourself to fast for one day when you can eat what you want the next day!

When you are eating on a fast day, be sure to get your small amount of calories from healthy foods that are high in fiber and protein to help keep your body shedding pounds. Do not eat carbohydrates on your fast days. Eat as many fresh, raw foods as possible on these days, as well. Drink water as much as possible, but you can also have coffee or tea as long as they are not filled with cream and sugar. Although you are welcome to drink healthy amounts of alcohol on the other five days, avoid alcoholic beverages on your fast days. Treat these two days a week as true "diet days!"

This method of dieting is proven to work. If you strictly follow the fasting program, you will lose roughly a pound a week. You are also sure to notice other benefits in your life, including lower blood pressure, better cholesterol, more even blood sugar levels, and improved digestive health. This is because your body exerts a great deal of effort and expends a lot of energy in digesting and expelling food. When you take two days off a week from eating, it allows your system to reset itself much more quickly. The body is able to spend more time and energy on other tasks, such as burning fat, restoring and maintaining cell growth, and keeping other processes moving along as they should.

Chances are, you have probably heard of the paleo style diet, and you may even already be following this simple weight loss lifestyle. Briefly, the paleo style diet focuses on eating only foods that early hunter-gatherers would have eaten. This means that if you could conceivably find, hunt, or grow a food item, you can eat it. A paleo style diet, therefore, includes all sorts of nuts, seeds, berries, fruits, vegetables, roots, spices, and meat. It does not included refined or processed foods such as bleached white sugar, bleached white flour, or anything with a chemical name on the list of ingredients. Basically, if you are completely certain of what goes into your food, you can easily follow this healthy and balanced way of eating.

The paleo style diet is easy to adapt to a 5:2 diet plan. Because this type of dieting is so healthy and so well-balanced, it is a great way to eat when you are not on your fasting days. You will be putting only quality food into your system, so that even if you are eating many calories on your non-fasting days, you will still be enjoying a healthy lifestyle. However, the paleo diet is not terribly restrictive, so you will not feel like you are dieting at all.

Too, when you are on your fasting days, you need to be sure that you are eating healthy, low-carb, high-protein meals that will keep your body functioning the best way possible. Anything on a paleo diet is sure to do that. Although you will have to watch your caloric intake, it is much easier to do that when you are eating healthy foods such as baked or roasted meats and fresh vegetables.

Combining the paleo diet with the 5:2 diet is the best way to lose weight fast and stay healthy. Enjoy weight loss of at least a pound a week by following these two diets put together.

SOFT BOILED EGG

Soft-boiled eggs can be surprisingly difficult to make, for those who have never given them a try before. However, for a protein-filled breakfast on your fasting days, you can't go wrong with a delicious soft-boiled egg. Just refrain from dipping bread in the egg if you're on a fasting day!

This recipe contains only 95 calories.

1 egg

3 cups water

1. Bring water to a boil over high heat in a small pot.

2. Gently place egg in boiling water.

3. Cover pot.

4. Reduce heat to low.

5. Simmer egg for 5 minutes.

6. Drain hot water from egg and rinse egg under ice cold water.

7. Gently crack top shell for easy scooping or peeling.

8. Serve in an egg cup.

SCRAMBLED EGGS WITH MUSHROOMS

Enjoy a morning breakfast that tastes hearty but doesn't have very many calories at all by preparing this simple fasting day recipe. If you have a handful of calories to spare from elsewhere in your day, you can top it with a few diced tomatoes.

This recipe contains only 110 calories.

1 egg

3 mushrooms

1. Black pepper to taste

2. Dice mushrooms into small pieces.

3. Crack egg into a small bowl.

4. Add 1 tbsp water.

5. Whisk egg and water together.

6. Add black pepper to taste and mushrooms.

7. Whisk to combine.

8. Pour into a skillet over medium-high heat.

9. Cook until egg starts to firm.

10. Scramble and continue to cook until egg is done.

11. Serve.

SPINACH OMELETTE

Eggs and spinach are both excellent sources of healthy proteins. Spinach is also chock full of iron, which your body needs.　You can't go wrong starting a fasting day with this simple and delicious breakfast.

This recipe contains only 110 calories.

1 egg

1 handful spinach

Black pepper to taste

Dried parsley to taste

1.	Break spinach into smaller pieces.

2.	Crack egg into a small bowl.

3.	Add 1 tbsp water.

4.	Whisk egg and water together.

5.	Add black pepper and dried parsley to taste.

6.	Whisk to combine.

7.	Pour into a skillet over medium-high heat.

8.	Cook until egg is done on the bottom.

9.	Add spinach to the top of the egg.

10.	Fold in half and cook until egg is done.

11.	Serve.

PORRIDGE

Although there are some carbs in porridge, they are the healthy type of carbs that release energy slowly over time after you consume them.   Therefore, a nice bowl of warm porridge to start a fasting day will keep you going strong until your next small meal.   Add cinnamon to help burn fat and not gain any extra calorie count.

This recipe contains only 100 calories.

1 cup rolled outs

1/2 cup water (or more, if you like soupier porridge)

Dried cinnamon to taste

1. In a small pot over medium heat, combine dry rolled oats, water, and dried cinnamon.

2. Stir continuously until mixture is boiling.

3. One boiling, reduce heat to low.

4. Simmer and continue stirring for 5 minutes.

5. Serve.

HAM OMELETTE

Although a ham omelette contains a few more calories than a spinach omelette does, it is an even better option if you are looking for a protein-packed breakfast to get you through a tough workout or the first part of your work day.

This recipe contains only 115 calories.

1 egg

1 tbsp water

1 slice deli ham

Black pepper to taste

1. Chop ham into small pieces.

2. Crack egg into a small bowl.

3. Add 1 tbsp water.

4. Whisk egg and water together.

5. Add black pepper to taste.

6. Whisk to combine.

7. Pour into a skillet over medium-high heat.

8. Cook until egg is done on the bottom.

9. Add diced ham to the top of the egg.

10. Fold in half and cook until egg is done.

11. Serve.

Chapter 4 - Fast Day Lunches

CHICKEN PITA POCKETS

This low calorie meal would make a great lunch even on a normal eating day! However, you can still enjoy one of these tasty pita pockets on a fast day without worrying about your caloric intake. Make extras for the kids to snack on after school!

This recipe contains only 160 calories.

1 tbsp low-fat yogurt

1 tsp tomato puree, unsalted

1 tsp curry paste

1 bag precooked diced unsalted chicken breasts

1 tsp olive oil

1 whole wheat pita pocket

Handful shredded lettuce

3 cherry tomatoes

1.   Halve cherry tomatoes.

2.   Combine yogurt, tomato puree, and curry paste.

3.   Add chicken to mixture and toss to coat thoroughly.

4.   Refrigerate for 15 minutes.

5.   Sauté marinated chicken over medium heat in 1 tsp olive oil in a large skillet until heated through.

6. Top pita pocket with lettuce, tomatoes, and chicken.

7. Serve.

SPRING SOUP

Make this soup ahead of time and enjoy it quickly on the go just by reheating it! It will keep for up to 2 weeks in the refrigerator. It is packed with vitamins, nutrients, and of course that vital protein and fiber you need on your fasting days.

This recipe contains only 160 calories.

2 cups chicken stock

1/2 onion

Handful baby carrots

1 stalk celery

1 leek

1 tbsp minced garlic

1 new potato

1/2 cup frozen peas

1 handful bok choy leaves

1. Peel and chop onion.

2. Cut baby carrots in half.

3. Dice celery and leek.

4. Quarter potato.

5. Bring chicken stock to a boil in a large pot on the stove.

6. Add onion, carrots, leek, and garlic, and boil again.

7. Add potatoes and simmer for 12 minutes.

8. Add peas and bok choy and simmer for 5 minutes.

9. Serve.

POTATOES AND SHOOTS

Get a few healthy carbs in the potatoes used in this perfect fasting lunchtime recipe. These are the good type of carbs that will help you burn energy well throughout the day, but won't make you feel exhausted immediately after eating them.

This recipe contains only 170 calories.

1 new potato

2 stalks asparagus

1 tbsp olive oil

1 tbsp lemon juice

2 green onions

1 egg

1 handful pea shoots

1 handful arugula

1. Finely chop green onions.

2. Hard or soft boil egg.

3. Bring a pot of water to a boil.

4. Add potato to boiling water.

5. Reduce heat to medium-low and simmer for 20 minutes.

6. Add asparagus to pot and simmer for 2 minutes more.

7. Drain and halve potatoes.

8. Mash potatoes into a bowl gently with a fork.

9. Combine oil and lemon juice and pour over potatoes.

10. Combine spring onion into mixture.

11. Arrange asparagus on a plate with potato mixture, egg halves, and pea shoots.

12. Arrange arugula around outside of plate.

13. Serve.

BEAN SALAD

Get plenty of fiber and protein both by loading up on beans with this yummy salad. You will feel fuller for much longer after eating this tasty dish. It is topped with a mustard dressing that will make you look forward to this fasting day meal!

This recipe contains only 180 calories.

handful frozen green beans

1/2 red onion

1 stalk celery

1/4 can cannellini beans

1/4 can borlotti beans

3 cherry tomatoes

2 tbsp mustard

1 tbsp honey

1 tbsp lemon juice

1 tbsp olive oil

1. Black pepper to taste

2. Peel and chop red onion.

3. Chop celery.

4. Rinse and drain all beans.

5. Cut cherry tomatoes in half.

6. Place green beans in a microwave-safe bowl with 2 tbsp water.

7. Cover with plastic wrap and pierce holes in wrap to vent.

8. Microwave on high for 2 minutes or until cooked to desired tenderness.

9. Add celery, beans, and tomatoes to green beans.

10. Combine mustard, honey, lemon juice, olive oil, and black pepper in a small jar.

11. Shake to combine well.

12. Top vegetables with dressing.

13. Serve.

TARKA DHAL

This recipe is a favorite Indian side dish that is often served with spicy chicken and bread. Enjoy it on its own for a yummy and unique lunch that is very low in calories.

This recipe contains only 140 calories.

1 cup dried yellow split peas

1 tbsp minced garlic

2 tsp dried ginger

1 tsp dried turmeric

2 tbsp olive oil

1/2 tsp dried cumin

1/2 onion

1 carrot

1 stalk celery

1/2 cucumber

1. Peel onion and cucumber and slice into strips.

2. Chop carrot and celery into dipping pieces.

3. Boil 2 cups water over high heat in a pot.

4. Add split peas, garlic, ginger, and turmeric and bring to a boil again.

5.	Cover and simmer for 45 minutes.

6.	Heat olive oil over medium heat in a skillet.

7.	Add cumin and onion to pan and cook for 15 minutes.

8.	When split pea mixture is smooth, top with onion mixture.

9.	Serve with vegetables for dipping.

STEAK SALAD

Incorporate yummy summertime vegetables into this tasty dish that won't tip your calories for the day. You'll barely realize you're eating a salad at all once you taste all the delicious flavors that combine in this great recipe!

This recipe contains only 180 calories.

2 tbsp olive oil

1 bag precooked diced steak strips, unsalted

1 orange

1 tsp Dijon mustard

Black pepper to taste

1 red onion

1/2 head white chicory

Handful of arugula

1.	Cut orange in half; peel and wedge one half and juice the other half.

2. Chop red onion into wedges.

3. Slice chicory into 2 pieces.

4. In a skillet over medium heat, sauté steak strips in 1 tsp olive oil.

5. In a separate skillet, boil orange juice.

6. Remove from heat and whisk in dijon mustard, 1 tsp olive oil, and black pepper to taste.

7. Toss onion and chicory in remaining olive oil.

8. Sauté onion and chicory for a few minutes.

9. Combine steak, orange wedges, and orange juice mixture.

10. Serve over arugula.

ARTICHOKE TORTILLA

Load up on protein with this tasty lunchtime take on a common breakfast recipe. The artichokes add tons of flavor to this already delicious dish. Add any other spices you may enjoy, as spices do not add any calories to your daily count.

This recipe contains only 110 calories.

5 artichoke hearts

1/2 large potato

1/2 small onion

1 egg

Fresh parsley to taste

1. Quarter artichoke hearts.

2. Peel potato and chop into cubes.

3. Peel and dice onion.

4. Chop parsley.

5. In a skillet over medium heat, dry sauté potato and onion for 10 minutes.

6. Beat egg well and season with fresh parsley.

7. Pour egg and parsley over potato mixture in skillet.

8. Add artichoke hearts to skillet.

9. Cook over medium heat until edges are firm.

10. Flip tortilla and cook other side over low heat for 5 minutes.

11. Cool and cut into wedges.

12. Serve.

MISO SOUP WITH CHICKEN

Mix up this recipe with just a few ingredients a few minutes of spare time on your hands. Check the Asian foods section of your local market for the miso paste, which is a healthy way to add flavor to any Asian-inspired dish.

This recipe contains only 130 calories.

1 miso paste sachet

1/2 chicken breast

1 tbsp minced garlic

1/2 tsp dried ginger

4 shiitake mushrooms

Savoy cabbage

1. Finely shred savoy cabbage.

2. Dice chicken breast into chunks.

3. Boil 1 pint of water on high heat and mix miso paste into boiling water.

4. Reduce heat to medium-low.

5. Add chicken, garlic, ginger, and mushrooms.

6. Cover and simmer for 10 minutes.

7. Add cabbage and simmer for 3 minutes.

8. Serve.

SHRIMP SALAD

Make your own salad dressing to ensure that you know exactly what is going into your body. By doing this, you can enjoy this delicious and incredibly healthy low-calorie lunch on a fasting day (or any day).

This recipe contains only 100 calories.

1 cucumber

1 handful baby spinach

2 tsp olive oil

3 raw shrimp

1 tbsp minced garlic

1 red chili pepper

1 tsp brown sugar

1 lime

1 tbsp fresh mint leaves

1. Remove seeds from chili pepper and dice pepper finely.

2. Juice lime.

3. Chop mint leaves.

4. Peel cucumber and dice finely.

5. Whisk together 1 tsp olive oil, minced garlic, diced chili pepper, brown sugar, juice from lime, and mint leaves in a small bowl.

6. Add cucumber to dressing and mix thoroughly to combine.

7. Top spinach with cucumber mixture.

8. In a small skillet over medium heat, cook shrimp in 1 tsp olive oil.

9. Cook for 4 minutes.

10. Top salad with shrimp.

11. Serve.

TOMATO SHRIMP

Enjoy a nice shrimpy soup with a yummy tomato sauce by preparing this recipe for one of your fasting day dinners. This one is low in calories but high in antioxidants. It's also full of amazing flavor that will surprise you with the first bite!

This recipe contains only 170 calories.

1 tbsp olive oil

1 tbsp minced garlic

Handful fresh parsley

3 cherry tomatoes

1 tbsp tomato paste

5 raw shrimp

Black pepper to taste

1. Peel shrimp.

2. In a large skillet, sauté garlic and parsley for 12 minutes over low heat in 1 tbsp olive oil.

3. Add cherry tomatoes and tomato paste and bring to a boil.

4. Reduce heat to low and simmer for 25 minutes.

5. Add shrimp and cook for 2 minutes.

6. Turn shrimp and cook for 2 minutes more.

7. Season with black pepper and parsley.

8. Serve.

EGGPLANT

This delicious dish is very easy to prepare and full of flavor. It is quite hearty, and will keep you feeling full for the rest of the night on your fasting day after dinner. If you have enough calories to spare, enjoy it with a slice of bread. Even without, it is very filling!

This recipe contains only 80 calories.

1 eggplant

1 tsp dried cumin

1/2 onion

1 tbsp minced garlic

1 tsp dried ginger

1 tomato

1 tsp turmeric

Black pepper to taste

1 tsp lemon juice

1. Chop onion and tomato.

2. Preheat oven to 350 degrees Fahrenheit.

3. Wash eggplant and prick with a knife to vent.

4. Cook eggplant for 20 minutes.

5. In a large skillet over high heat, cook onion and cumin for 10 minutes.

6. Add garlic and ginger and cook for 1 minute.

7. Add tomato, turmeric, and black pepper, and cook for 2 minutes.

8. Scoop out the insides of the eggplant and mix with lemon juice.

9. Add eggplant and lemon juice mash to mixture in skillet.

10. Cook for 10 minutes on low.

11. Stuff mixture into eggplant skin.

12. Serve.

CHOW MEIN

Make the chow mein noodles for this dish out of spaghetti squash to keep your calorie count low and your paleo diet on track at the same time. You won't even realize you're eating on a diet when you chow down on this filling dinner!

This recipe contains only 170 calories.

1 tbsp olive oil

5 oyster mushrooms

1 red bell pepper

Handful frozen broccoli

1 carrot

1 tbsp apple cider vinegar

1 tbsp oyster sauce

1 spaghetti squash

1. Slice mushrooms.

2. Remove seeds from bell pepper and slice.

3. Dice carrot.

4. Cut spaghetti squash in half and remove seeds and guts.

5. Place squash halves on a microwave safe baking dish with 1 tbsp of water.

6. Cook in the microwave for 4 minute per pound of squash, or until meat of squash can be pierced easily with a fork.

7. Remove and let cool.

8. Use a fork to shred squash innards into long stringy noodles.

9. In a large skillet, heat olive oil over medium heat.

10. Add mushrooms, bell pepper, broccoli, and carrot and cook for 3 minutes.

11. Add apple cider vinegar and soy sauce and cook for 1 minute.

12. Add spaghetti squash noodles and stir to mix thoroughly and heat through.

13. Serve.

SQUASH TORTILLA

Enjoy the autumnal taste of butternut squash mixed with a great deal of protein in the egg and spinach. You will feel full and healthy with all of the nutrients packed into this low calorie meal.

This recipe contains only 190 calories.

1 butternut squash

1 egg

2 tbsp skim milk

1 tsp dijon mustard

Handful baby spinach leaves

Black pepper to taste

1. Peel squash, remove seeds, and dice finely.

2. Boil water in a pot on the stove.

3. Add squash and reduce heat to medium.

4. Cook for 15 minutes and drain.

5. In a large bowl, combine eggs, milk, mustard, and black pepper.

6. In a large skillet, fry squash for 2 minutes.

7. Add spinach and stir fry for 2 minutes.

8. Cover with egg mixture.

9. Stir and cook on low for 10 minutes until the bottom is cooked.

10. Flip and cook the other side.

11. Serve.

RATATOUILLE

This recipe is incredibly filling despite being made entirely of vegetables. You won't have a chance to miss meat while you are devouring this yummy tomato based dinner.

This recipe contains only 150 calories.

1 red bell pepper

1 eggplant

1 zucchini

1 red onion

1 tomato

1 tbsp dried oregano

1 tbsp olive oil

1 tbsp minced garlic

Can chopped tomatoes

1. Remove seeds from red bell pepper and cut into large chunks.

2. Slice eggplant thickly.

3. Dice red onion and zucchini into chunks.

4. Halve tomato.

5. Combine all ingredients into a slow cooker, with the canned chopped tomatoes on top.

6. Stir well to combine thoroughly.

7. Cook on low setting for 3 hours.

8. Serve.

SPICED SQUASH

These veggies will be full of amazing flavor when you cook them in this Moroccan inspired dish. The chickpeas, as an added bonus, are a source of healthy fats that will keep you feeling full.

This recipe contains only 150 calories.

2 tbsp olive oil

1 butternut squash

1 onion

1 parsnip

1/2 head cauliflower

1 carrot

1 red bell pepper

1 tbsp ground cumin

1 tbsp ground turmeric

Can chopped tomatoes

1 cube chicken stock

Can chickpeas

1. Peel squash, remove seeds, and cut into large chunks.

2. Peel onion and parsnip and cut into chunks.

3. Break florets from cauliflower.

4. Peel and slice carrot.

5. Remove seeds from bell pepper and chop.

6. Drain and rinse chickpeas.

7. Cook onion in olive oil in a large skillet for 5 minutes.

8. Add parsnip, cauliflower, carrot, and bell pepper to onion and cook for 5 minutes more.

9. Add ground cumin and turmeric and cook for 2 minutes more.

10. Add chopped tomatoes, chicken stock, and chickpeas and bring to a boil.

11. Pour into slow cooker and cook on high for 3 hours.

12. Serve.

FISH BURGER

Serve this burger on a bed of lettuce in place of a bun to keep it under your calorie count for the day. It is a delicious way to get the healthy omega-3s found in fish while treating yourself to a tasty dinner!

This recipe contains only 140 calories.

1 can tuna

2 tbsp fresh parsley

1 tbsp capers

1 tbsp olive oil

Romaine lettuce

1. Chop fresh parsley.

2. Combine parsley, tuna, and capers, and form into burger patties by hand.

3. Fry patties over medium heat in olive oil in a small skillet for 3 minutes per side.

4. Serve over romaine.

BALTI

Although this recipe is usually served over rice, leaving off the rice makes it well below your calorie count for a fasting day. This also puts this recipe solidly in the realm of paleo dieting, by eliminating the grain.

This recipe contains only 130 calories.

1 tbsp olive oil

1 onion

3 tbsp curry paste

1 parsnip

1 butternut squash

Can chopped tomatoes

1 cup chicken stock

1/2 head cauliflower

1. Dice onion and parsnips.

2. Peel squash and cut into cubes.

3. Remove florets from cauliflower.

4. Cook onion in olive oil for 5 minutes in a large skillet.

5. Add curry paste and cook for 1 minute more.

6. Add parsnip, squash, tomatoes, and chicken stock and bring to a boil.

7. Reduce heat to low and simmer for 10 minutes.

8. Add cauliflower and cook for 5 minutes.

9. Serve.

MEDITERRANEAN CHILI

Pack a bowl with these tasty vegetables and feel great for eating a healthy, low-calorie meal that doesn't make you feel bloated or fatigued afterward. The kidney beans will give you lots of energy, and the lack of rice keeps it paleo friendly.

This recipe contains only 190 calories.

1 tbsp olive oil

1 onion

1 yellow bell pepper

1 eggplant

1 zucchini

2 tbsp chili powder

5 cherry tomatoes

1 can kidney beans

Handful baby spinach

1. Dice red onion, bell pepper, zucchini, and eggplant.

2. Drain kidney beans.

3. In a large skillet, cook onion, bell pepper, zucchini, and eggplant in chili powder and olive oil over medium heat for 10 minutes.

4. Add cherry tomatoes and kidney beans.

5. Reduce heat to low and simmer for 15 minutes.

6. Add spinach and stir to mix thoroughly.

7. Serve.

THAI CHICKEN

Although this recipe is slightly higher in caloric content than the others listed here, it can still work beautifully as a fasting day dinner when you have had lower calorie meals the rest of the day. Eat it to feel full and energetic!

This recipe contains only 280 calories.

1 tbsp olive oil

1 chicken breast

1 yellow bell pepper

1 can coconut milk

1 cup cold water

1 tbsp curry paste

1 tbsp fish sauce

1 tbsp dried basil

1. Slice chicken breast thinly.

2. Remove seeds from bell pepper and slice thinly.

3. In a large skillet over medium heat, stir-fry chicken and bell pepper in olive oil for 1 minute.

4. Pour over coconut milk, water, curry paste, and fish sauce and bring to a boil.

5. Reduce heat to low and simmer for 5 minutes.

6. Add basil and stir.

7. Cook for 2 minutes more.

8. Serve.

MOROCCAN TOMATOES

This is a unique dish inspired by Moroccan flavors and modified to fit snugly into a paleo friendly and low calorie diet. Enjoy all the protein of eggs with all the flavor of asparagus in this delicious and interesting soupy dinner. Tomatoes add much-needed antioxidants.

This recipe contains only 220 calories.

1 tbsp olive oil

2 stalks asparagus

1 tbsp minced garlic

1 tomato

1 egg

1 tsp dried cumin

1. Halve asparagus.

2. Slice tomato thickly.

3. Cook asparagus in olive oil in a large skillet over medium heat for 2 minutes.

4. Add garlic and tomato and cook for 2 minutes more.

5. Move vegetables to the side of the pan and break two eggs into the empty space.

6. Cover and cook for 5 minutes.

7. Season with cumin.

8. Serve.

Chapter 6 - One Month of Fasting Day Suggestions

While following a 5:2 diet, it is important to remember the basics of the diet itself:

Remember that for five days out of the week, you can eat whatever you want.

Remember that you do not have to eat and fast in the 3-on, 1-off, 2-on, 1-off pattern listed below. This is simply a guideline, and you can choose which days of the week are best for you to fast. You can also change the days each week, as long as you are fasting for two days out of seven.

When combining the 5:2 diet with a paleo diet, make sure that the foods you eat on your normal eating days fall into the paleo dietary restrictions.

For example, on your normal eating days, eat plenty of meat, vegetables, fruits, spices, eggs, and dairy, but do not eat salt, refined sugar, grains, or any processed foods. TIP: Use honey for a sweetener!

If you come in under your calorie limit for the fasting days (500 calories for women and 600 calories for men), be sure to eat a low calorie snack to make up the difference. Eating too few calories will actually cause you to gain weight.

Good paleo friendly low calorie snacks include Greek yogurt, a boiled egg, a piece of fruit, or fresh vegetables.

On fasting days, you can easily still eat a paleo diet by following the plan outlined below.

Week One

Days 1-3

Eat whatever you like that fits into the paleo style dietary restrictions outlined above.

Day 4 - Total Calories: 445

Breakfast - Soft-Boiled Egg - 95 calories

Lunch - Chicken Pita Pockets - 160 calories

Dinner - Mediterranean Chili - 190 calories

Shopping List

1 egg

Low-fat yogurt

Tomato puree

Curry paste

1 bag precooked diced unsalted chicken breasts

Olive oil

1 whole wheat pita pocket

Shredded lettuce

Cherry tomatoes

1 onion

1 yellow bell pepper

1 eggplant

1 zucchini

Chili powder

1 can kidney beans

Baby spinach

Days 5-6

Eat whatever you like that fits into the paleo style dietary restrictions outlined above.

Day 7 - Total Calories: 400

Breakfast - Scrambled Eggs with Mushrooms - 110 calories

Lunch - Spring Soup - 160 calories

Dinner - Balti - 130 calories

Shopping List

1 egg

3 mushrooms

Chicken stock

2 onions

Handful baby carrots

1 stalk celery

1 leek

Minced garlic

1 new potato

Frozen peas

Bok choy

Olive oil

Curry paste

1 parsnip

1 butternut squash

Canned chopped tomatoes

Chicken stock

Cauliflower

Week Two

Days 8-10

Eat whatever you like that fits into the paleo style dietary restrictions outlined above.

Day 11 - Total Calories: 405

Breakfast - Soft-Boiled Egg - 95 calories

Lunch - Potatoes and Shoots - 170 calories

Dinner - Fish Burger - 140 calories

Shopping List

2 eggs

1 new potato

2 stalks asparagus

Olive oil

Lemon juice

2 green onions

1 handful pea shoots

1 handful arugula

1 can tuna

Fresh parsley

Capers

Romaine lettuce

Days 12-13

Eat whatever you like that fits into the paleo style dietary restrictions outlined above.

Day 14 - Total Calories: 440 calories

Breakfast - Spinach Omelette - 110 calories

Lunch - Bean Salad - 180 calories

Dinner - Ratatouille - 150 calories

Shopping List

1 egg

1 handful spinach

Dried parsley

Frozen green beans

2 red onions

1 stalk celery

Canned cannellini beans

Canned borlotti beans

Cherry tomatoes

Mustard

Honey

Lemon juice

Olive oil

Canned chopped tomatoes

Minced garlic

Dried oregano

1 tomato

1 zucchini

1 eggplant

1 red bell pepper

Week Three

Days 15-17

Eat whatever you like that fits into the paleo style dietary restrictions outlined above.

Day 18 - Total Calories: 465

Breakfast - Soft-Boiled Egg - 95 calories

Lunch - Steak Salad - 180 calories

Dinner - Squash Tortilla - 190 calories

Shopping List

2 eggs

1 bag precooked diced steak strips

Olive oil

1 orange

Dijon musard

red onion

1 head white chicory

Handful of arugula

1 butternut squash

Skim milk

Handful of baby spinach

Days 19-20

Eat whatever you like that fits into the paleo style dietary restrictions outlined above.

Day 21 - Total Calories: 380

Breakfast - Porridge - 100 calories

Lunch - Artichoke Tortilla - 110 calories

Dinner - Chow Mein - 170 calories

Shopping List

1 cup rolled oats

Dried cinnamon

Artichoke hearts

Large potato

Small onion

1 egg

Fresh parsley

Olive oil

5 oyster mushrooms

1 red bell pepper

Handful frozen broccoli

1 carrot

Apple cider vinegar

Oyster sauce

Spaghetti squash

Week Four

Days 22-24

Eat whatever you like that fits into the paleo style dietary restrictions outlined above.

Day 25 - Total Calories: 305

Breakfast - Soft-Boiled Egg - 95 calories

Lunch - Miso Soup with Chicken - 130 calories

Dinner - Eggplant - 80 calories

Shopping List

1 egg

1 miso paste sachet

1 chicken breast

Minced garlic

Dried ginger

4 shiitake mushrooms

Savoy cabbage

1 eggplant

Dried cumin

1 onion

1 tomato

Turmeric

Days 26-27

Eat whatever you like that fits into the paleo style dietary restrictions outlined above.

Day 28 - Total Calories: 385

Breakfast - Ham Omelette - 115 calories

Lunch - Shrimp Salad - 100 calories

Dinner - Tomato Shrimp - 170 calories

Shopping List

1 egg

1 slice deli ham

1 cucumber

Handful baby spinach

olive oil

8 raw shrimp

Minced garlic

1 red chili pepper

Brown sugar

1 lime

Fresh mint leaves

Handful fresh parsley

Cherry tomatoes

Tomato paste

Conclusion

Thank you again for downloading this book!

I hope this book was able to help you to understand how easy it can be to lose weight on a 5:2 paleo combination diet.

The next step is to start cooking!

OTHER RECOMMENDED BOOKS

Paleo for Beginners: Essentials to Get Started with the Paleo Diet (Click to on title go to Amazon link)

Book Description

The Paleo diet is not just another fad diet; it is the diet humans were designed to eat. Also known as the Primal diet, the Caveman diet, and the Stone Age diet, the Paleo diet focuses on low-carb, high-protein meals, and removes all processed foods.

Paleo for Beginners will show you how to adopt a Paleo lifestyle in order to feel healthy, lose weight, and increase your energy level. With Paleo for Beginners, start enjoying the best health of your life today--all while losing weight and decreasing your odds of diabetes, hypertension, heart disease, cancer, osteoporosis, and many other modern health maladies.

This is A Preview Of What You'll Learn...

Successfully make the transition to a Paleo lifestyle with a 7-day, step-by-step plan for beginners

Set yourself up for success with the Paleo shopping guide and a list of 117 Paleo-recommended foods (and an extensive list of what food items you should avoid).

Enjoy Paleo-friendly versions of 99 mouthwatering recipes for every meal. Recipes include Eggs Benedict Paleo Style, High-Protein Grain-Free Burgers, Chicken Avocado Wraps, and Paleo Waffles.

OTHER BOOKS FROM J.S. WEST

Amazon
Kindle

Click Images
for Links

*go to
J.S. West
Author Page*

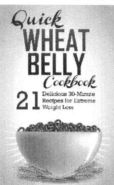

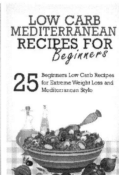

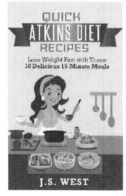

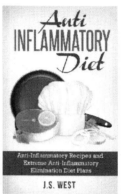

LOW CARB CROCK POT *Cookbook*

25 Quick and Easy Slow Cooker Paleo Diet Recipes for Busy People to Lose Weight Fast

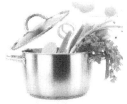

PALEO LOW CARB *COOKBOOK*

50 Essential Low Carb Paleo Recipes for Weight Loss and Paleo Style Life

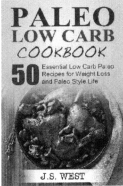

J.S. WEST

LOW CARB PALEO *COOKBOOK*

25 Delicious Low Budget Paleo Recipes for Low-Carb Weight Loss

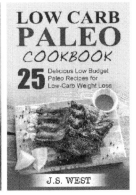

J.S. WEST

LOW CARB SLOW COOKER PALEO RECIPES *for Beginners*

25 Beginners Low Carb Slow Cooker Recipes for Extreme Weight Loss and Paleo Style

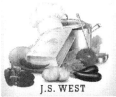

J.S. WEST

13-Day GREEN SMOOTHIE *Cleanse*

Extreme Weight Loss and Paleo Style

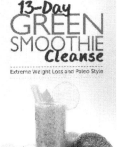

J.S. WEST

Amazon
Kindle

Click Images for Links

go to
J.S. West
Author Page

OTHER BOOKS FROM J.S. WEST

Paleo Diet: Paleo Low Carb Slow Cooker Recipes for Beginners - Weight Loss and Paleo Style (Click to on title go to Amazon link)

Book Description

Many people in today's society are unhappy with the state of their health and wellbeing. Some want to lose weight; others have frequent stomach upset that interferes with daily life. Still others have skin problems or emotional irritability that can be easily related to eating foods that are not healthy for the body.

Early man did not have these kinds of problems. "Cavemen," as most people refer to them, ate what they could hunt, find, and pluck from the trees. They were fit and not overweight, and were generally quite healthy. The paleo diet is a recent lifestyle based on the overall food consumption of the early man, and the trend is quickly gaining popularity. It has many proven and documented health benefits, including weight loss, improved digestive systems, and increased energy levels without the use of caffeine.

This book should serve as a helpful resource for anyone looking to get started on a paleo diet. The first part of the book will explain, briefly, the definition of a paleo diet, what can and cannot be eaten when following a paleo diet, and the items most necessary to keep in stock in a paleo-friendly kitchen. The rest of the book will be devoted to paleo recipes that can be cooked either completely or almost completely in a slow cooker. These recipes will be simple, but tasty, and will be perfect options for those who are just beginning to learn about paleo dieting. A slow cooker is a very easy and affordable option for cooking new recipes and starting a new diet, since the food can be prepared ahead of time and kept warm safely for hours.

This is A Preview Of What You'll Learn...

You will be excited and ready to try eating "like a caveman" in your own life. The health and wellness benefits will be incredible!

an understanding of the paleo diet and its benefits

what ingredients you need to set up a paleo kitchen

easy and delicious paleo slow cooker recipes

sample paleo meal plans

and much, much more!

[JOIN FOR FREE]

If you liked this book I'm sure that YOU will LIKE my other books as well.
Join my mailing list and get updates on FREE deals, new releases, bonus content and many others.
Click Here To Join for FREE

THANK YOU!!

Thank you again for downloading our book!

I hope this book was able to help you to achieve your health goals.

The next step is to apply what you've learned in this book and try out the great recipes provided.

If you enjoyed this book, please share your thoughts and leave a review on Amazon. Your feedback is important to us in order to improve the quality of the book.

CLICK HERE to LEAVE REVIEW

Good luck!

Printed in Great Britain
by Amazon